THE
ENDOMORPH
Diet Cookbook
For BEGINNERS

Unlock Your Body's Potential With 20 Quick And Easy Meal Plans To Achieve Sustainable Weight Loss And Transform Your Endomorph Body

MARIYAM MOHL

Copyright © 2023 by Mariyam Mohl

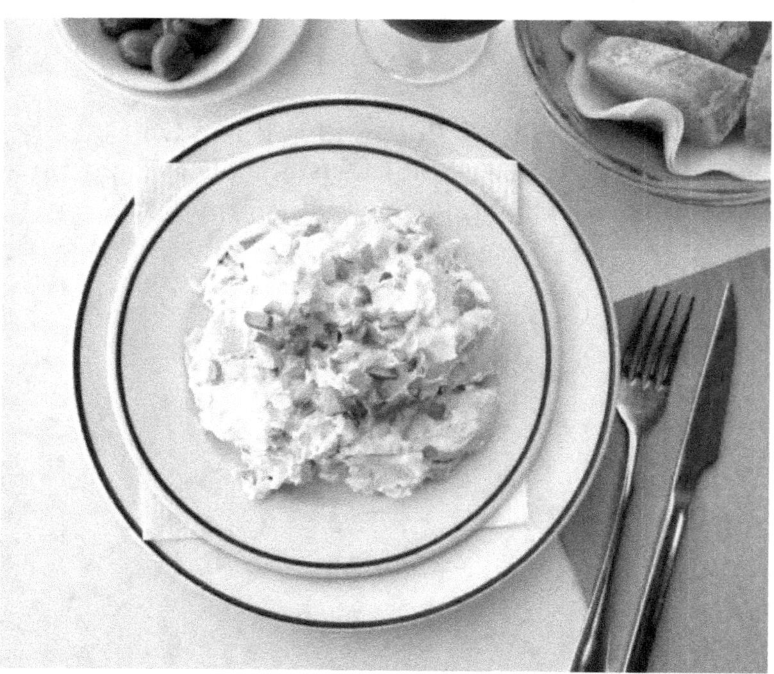

TABLE OF CONTENT

INTRODUCTION

Allow me to introduce you to "The Endomorph Diet Cookbook: A Fast and Easy Way to a Healthier You"—your key to discovering the details of a diet designed especially for those with an endomorph body type. This is your road map to a happier, better life, not just another recipe.

We recognize that selecting the best diet plan might be difficult in a world full of innumerable regimens and intricate recipes. For this reason, in addition to being tasty, our cookbook is also very simple to follow and quick to make. With "The Endomorph Diet Cookbook," you'll be well on your way to being a happier, healthier version of yourself.

1. Simplicity and Speed: We understand that you have a busy life and that cooking can seem like a difficult undertaking. Our recipes are meant to be easy to follow, uncomplicated, and quick. These dishes are your quick and simple fix; there's no need to spend hours in the kitchen.

2. Customized for You: Endomorphs, you should have a diet that honors the uniqueness of your body. This cookbook was created with your body's needs in mind. Personalized sustenance is here to replace generic diets.

3. Long-Term Results: Ignore yo-yo dieting and fast remedies. These simple, common meals will show you how to reach and keep your weight and health objectives in a sustainable way.

4. Energy On Demand: Bid adieu to the noon fall in energy. Our recipes are thoughtfully designed to give you a steady flow of energy throughout the day, enabling you to face life's obstacles with vigor.

5. Enhanced Well-Being: Experience a change from inside. Our quick and simple meals are designed to enhance your general health. You'll experience improved digestion, happier, more stable moods, and greater self-assurance.

6. Indulge Your Taste Buds: Dietary dull and boring fare is over. You're taken on a culinary adventure through the pages of our cookbook. As you set off on a gastronomic adventure that supports your health objectives, your taste buds will be grateful.

7. Savor the Journey: Following a diet ought to be enjoyable rather than laborious. "The Endomorph Diet Cookbook" enables you to enjoy feeding your body with scrumptious yet healthful cuisine.

This book is the solution if you're looking for a quicker, simpler, and more pleasurable way to become healthier. The advantages are obvious:

ease of use, quickness, and a menu customized to your endomorph requirements. It's time to include wellness into your life in a tasty and easy way. Welcome to a new phase in your quest to become a better, happier version of yourself.

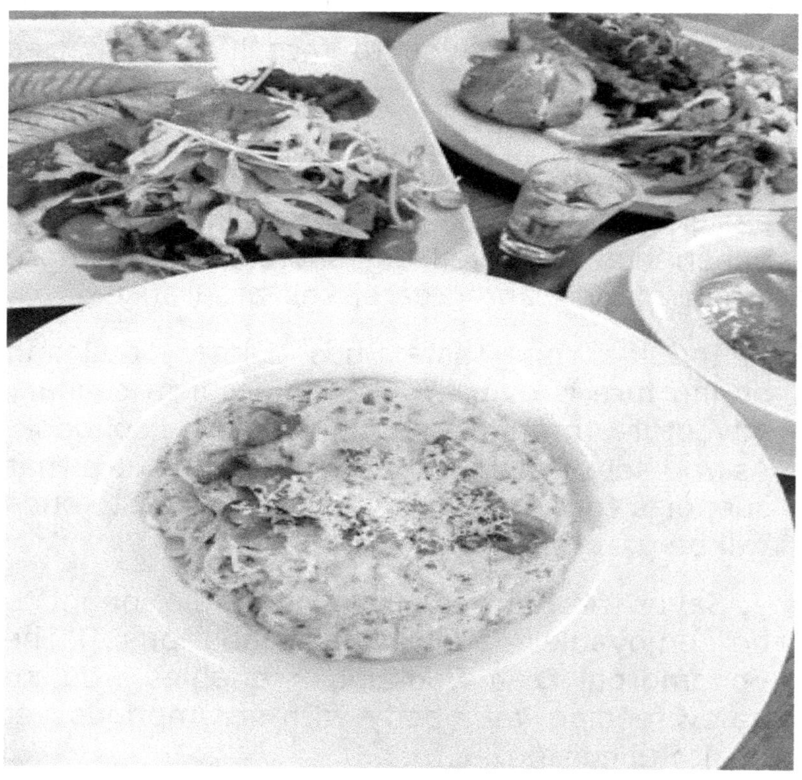

Grilled Chicken with Quinoa Salad

Ingredients:

For the Grilled Chicken:

- 2 boneless, skinless chicken breasts
- 2 tablespoons olive oil
- 1 teaspoon dried oregano
- 1 teaspoon paprika
- Salt and pepper to taste

For the Quinoa Salad:

- 1 cup quinoa, rinsed and drained
- 2 cups water or chicken broth
- 1 cucumber, diced
- 1 red bell pepper, diced
- 1/2 red onion, finely chopped
- 1/4 cup fresh parsley, chopped
- 1/4 cup feta cheese, crumbled (optional)
- Juice of 1 lemon
- 2 tablespoons extra-virgin olive oil
- Salt and pepper to taste

Instructions:

Grilled Chicken:

1. In a bowl, combine olive oil, dried oregano, paprika, salt, and pepper to create a marinade.

2. Place the chicken breasts in a zip-top bag or a shallow dish and pour the marinade over them.

3. Seal the bag or cover the dish and marinate the chicken in the refrigerator for at least 30 minutes, or ideally a few hours.

4. Preheat your grill to medium-high heat.

5. Remove the chicken from the marinade and grill for about 6-8 minutes per side, or until the internal temperature reaches 165°F (75°C) and the chicken is no longer pink in the center.

6. Let the chicken rest for a few minutes before slicing it into thin strips.

Quinoa Salad:

1. In a medium saucepan, bring 2 cups of water or chicken broth to a boil. Add quinoa, reduce heat to low, cover, and simmer for about 15 minutes, or until the

liquid is absorbed and the quinoa is fluffy. Remove from heat and let it cool.

2. In a large mixing bowl, combine the cooked quinoa, diced cucumber, red bell pepper, chopped red onion, and fresh parsley.

3. In a separate small bowl, whisk together the lemon juice and extra-virgin olive oil. Season with salt and pepper.

4. Pour the dressing over the quinoa salad and toss to combine.

5. If desired, top the salad with crumbled feta cheese.

6. Serve the grilled chicken strips on top of the quinoa salad.

Benefits:

- High in protein: Grilled chicken is a lean source of protein, essential for muscle development and repair.

- Balanced carbohydrates: Quinoa is a whole grain with complex carbohydrates, providing long-lasting energy.

- Rich in fiber: The salad's vegetables and quinoa are high in fiber, aiding in digestion.

- Healthy fats: Olive oil in the dressing provides heart-healthy monounsaturated fats.

- Vitamins and minerals: The salad is packed with vitamins, minerals, and antioxidants from the vegetables and herbs.

Applications:

- This dish is perfect for a healthy lunch or dinner option.

- You can prepare it in advance for meal prepping.

- Serve it at barbecues or picnics as a nutritious alternative.

- Customize the salad by adding other vegetables like cherry tomatoes, olives, or avocado.

- Adjust the seasonings and ingredients according to your taste and dietary preferences.

Sweet Potato and Black Bean Chili

Ingredients:

- 2 tablespoons olive oil
- 1 onion, chopped
- 2 cloves garlic, minced
- 1 large sweet potato, peeled and diced
- 1 red bell pepper, diced
- 1 can (15 oz) black beans, drained and rinsed
- 1 can (15 oz) diced tomatoes
- 2 cups vegetable broth
- 2 teaspoons chili powder
- 1 teaspoon ground cumin
- 1/2 teaspoon smoked paprika
- Salt and pepper to taste
- Fresh cilantro for garnish (optional)
- Lime wedges for serving (optional)

Instructions:

1. In a large pot, heat the olive oil over medium heat.

2. Add the chopped onion and minced garlic, sauté until fragrant and the onion is translucent, about 2-3 minutes.

3. Stir in the sweet potato and red bell pepper. Cook for another 5 minutes, stirring occasionally, until the sweet potato starts to soften.

4. Add the black beans, diced tomatoes (with their juice), vegetable broth, chili powder, ground cumin, smoked paprika, salt, and pepper. Stir to combine.

5. Bring the mixture to a boil, then reduce the heat to low, cover, and simmer for 20-25 minutes, or until the sweet potatoes are tender.

6. Taste and adjust the seasonings as needed.

7. Serve the sweet potato and black bean chili hot, garnished with fresh cilantro and lime wedges if desired.

Benefits:

- Nutrient-rich: Sweet potatoes are a great source of vitamins and fiber, while black beans provide protein and fiber.

- Low in fat: This chili is relatively low in fat, making it a healthy option.

- Vegetarian and vegan-friendly: Perfect for those following plant-based diets.

- High in antioxidants: The ingredients, like sweet potatoes and red bell peppers, are rich in antioxidants.

- Fiber-rich: Black beans and vegetables add a good amount of dietary fiber, aiding digestion.

Applications:

- Serve as a comforting and hearty main dish, especially on cool evenings.

- It's perfect for batch cooking and meal prep. Make a large batch and freeze for later.

- You can customize the spice level to suit your taste by adjusting the amount of chili powder.

- Top with your favorite chili toppings such as sour cream, shredded cheese, or diced avocado.

- Pair with cornbread, tortilla chips, or a side salad for a complete meal.

- Make it for potlucks, gatherings, or as a meatless option for chili cook-offs.

Baked Salmon with Asparagus

Ingredients:

- 2 salmon fillets (6-8 ounces each)
- 1 bunch of fresh asparagus
- 2 tablespoons olive oil
- 2 cloves garlic, minced
- 1 lemon, sliced
- 1 teaspoon dried dill (or fresh if available)
- Salt and pepper to taste
- Lemon wedges and fresh dill for garnish (optional)

Instructions:

1. Preheat your oven to 375°F (190°C).

2. Wash and trim the asparagus by snapping off the woody ends.

3. In a mixing bowl, combine olive oil, minced garlic, dried dill, salt, and pepper. Mix well.

4. Place the salmon fillets on a baking sheet lined with parchment paper or lightly greased. Drizzle some of the olive oil mixture over the salmon.

5. Arrange the asparagus around the salmon on the baking sheet, and drizzle the remaining olive oil mixture over the asparagus. Toss the asparagus to coat evenly.

6. Lay lemon slices over the salmon fillets.

7. Bake in the preheated oven for about 12-15 minutes or until the salmon flakes easily with a fork and the asparagus is tender.

8. Optionally, garnish with fresh dill and serve with lemon wedges.

Benefits:

- High in Omega-3 fatty acids: Salmon is rich in heart-healthy Omega-3s.

- Lean protein source: Salmon provides a good source of high-quality protein.

- Nutrient-rich: Asparagus is packed with vitamins, minerals, and fiber.

- Low in saturated fat: This dish is relatively low in unhealthy saturated fats.

- Garlic and dill add flavor without excess salt.

Applications:

- Ideal for a nutritious and elegant dinner option.

- Great for special occasions and entertaining guests.

- Suitable for a quick weeknight dinner since it's easy to prepare.

- Serve with a side of quinoa, rice, or a fresh salad for a well-rounded meal.

- You can customize the seasonings or add your favorite herbs and spices.

- Leftovers can be flaked and used in salads, sandwiches, or wraps.

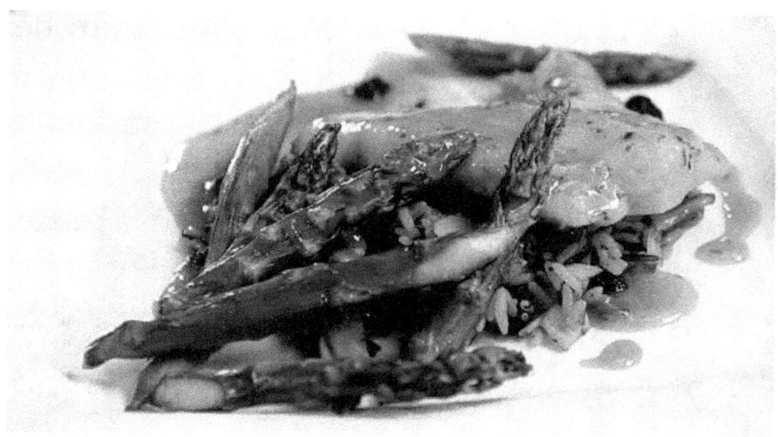

Turkey and Spinach Stuffed Peppers

Ingredients:

For the Stuffed Peppers:

- 4 large bell peppers (any color)
- 1 pound ground turkey
- 1 small onion, finely chopped
- 2 cloves garlic, minced
- 1 cup fresh spinach, chopped
- 1 cup cooked quinoa or brown rice
- 1 can (14 oz) diced tomatoes, drained
- 1 teaspoon dried oregano
- Salt and pepper to taste
- 1 cup shredded cheese (optional, for topping)

For the Tomato Sauce:

- 1 can (14 oz) tomato sauce
- 1 teaspoon Italian seasoning
- Salt and pepper to taste

Instructions:

Stuffed Peppers:

1. Preheat your oven to 375°F (190°C).

2. Cut the tops off the bell peppers, remove the seeds, and set them aside.

3. In a large skillet, cook the ground turkey over medium heat, breaking it apart as it cooks. When it's no longer pink, remove it from the skillet and set it aside.

4. In the same skillet, add a little olive oil if needed and sauté the chopped onion until translucent, about 2-3 minutes. Add minced garlic and cook for another minute.

5. Add the cooked turkey back into the skillet along with the chopped spinach, cooked quinoa (or rice), diced tomatoes, dried oregano, salt, and pepper. Cook for a few minutes until the spinach wilts and the mixture is well combined.

6. Stuff the bell peppers with the turkey and spinach mixture, packing them tightly.

7. Place the stuffed peppers in a baking dish.

8. If desired, top each stuffed pepper with shredded cheese.

9. Cover the baking dish with foil and bake for 30-35 minutes, or until the peppers are tender.

Tomato Sauce:

1. While the stuffed peppers are baking, prepare the tomato sauce. In a saucepan, combine the tomato sauce, Italian seasoning, salt, and pepper. Heat over low heat until warmed.

2. Serve the stuffed peppers with the tomato sauce drizzled over them.

Benefits:

- High in protein: Turkey provides lean protein for muscle health.

- Rich in fiber: Bell peppers, spinach, and quinoa (or brown rice) offer dietary fiber for digestion.

- Nutrient-packed: Spinach is a good source of vitamins and minerals.

- Low in saturated fat: This dish is relatively low in unhealthy saturated fats.

- A balanced meal with vegetables, protein, and whole grains.

Applications:

- Perfect for a wholesome and filling dinner option.

- Make it ahead and reheat for a quick weekday meal.

- Suitable for a family dinner or a meal to share with friends.

- Customize the stuffing with your favorite vegetables and spices.

- Serve as a main dish with a side salad or as part of a larger meal.

- Leftover filling can be used for stuffed zucchinis, tomatoes, or even in a burrito.

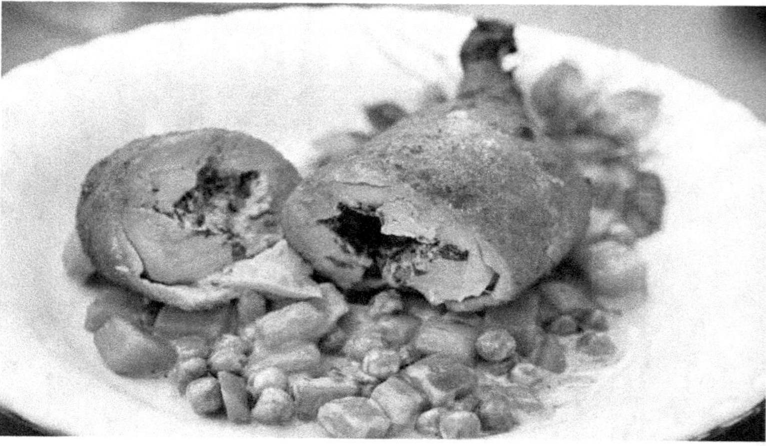

Lentil and Vegetable Stir-Fry

Ingredients:

- 1 cup dried green or brown lentils
- 2 cups water
- 2 tablespoons vegetable oil (for stir-frying)
- 1 onion, thinly sliced
- 2 cloves garlic, minced
- 1 red bell pepper, thinly sliced
- 1 yellow bell pepper, thinly sliced
- 1 zucchini, thinly sliced
- 1 cup broccoli florets
- 1 carrot, thinly sliced
- 1/4 cup low-sodium soy sauce
- 1 teaspoon ginger, minced (or ginger paste)
- 1 teaspoon sesame oil
- 1 tablespoon cornstarch (dissolved in 2 tablespoons of water)
- Salt and pepper to taste
- Optional garnishes: chopped green onions, sesame seeds

Instructions:

1. Rinse the lentils under cold water, then combine them with 2 cups of water in a medium saucepan. Bring to a boil, reduce heat, cover, and simmer for about 20-25 minutes, or until the lentils are tender but not mushy. Drain any excess water.

2. In a large skillet or wok, heat the vegetable oil over medium-high heat.

3. Add the sliced onion and garlic, and stir-fry for 2-3 minutes until they begin to soften and become fragrant.

4. Add the bell peppers, zucchini, broccoli, and carrot slices to the skillet. Stir-fry for about 5-7 minutes, or until the vegetables are tender-crisp.

5. In a small bowl, combine the soy sauce, minced ginger, sesame oil, and dissolved cornstarch. Mix well.

6. Pour the sauce mixture over the stir-fried vegetables and toss to coat. Continue cooking for a few minutes until the sauce thickens.

7. Stir in the cooked lentils and cook for an additional 2-3 minutes until everything is well combined and heated through.

8. Season with salt and pepper to taste.

9. Garnish with chopped green onions and sesame seeds if desired.

Benefits:

- Rich in plant-based protein: Lentils provide a good source of vegetarian protein.

- Low in saturated fat: This dish is relatively low in unhealthy saturated fats.

- High in fiber: Lentils and vegetables contribute dietary fiber for digestion.

- Nutrient-packed: The variety of colorful vegetables offer a range of vitamins and minerals.

- Suitable for vegetarians and vegans.

Applications:

- A healthy and balanced vegetarian or vegan main course.

- Make it for a quick and flavorful weeknight dinner.

- Customize the vegetables to your liking or based on what's in season.

- You can adjust the level of spiciness by adding chili sauce or red pepper flakes.

- Serve it over brown rice, quinoa, or whole wheat noodles for a complete meal.

- Leftovers can be enjoyed cold as a salad or reheated for another meal.

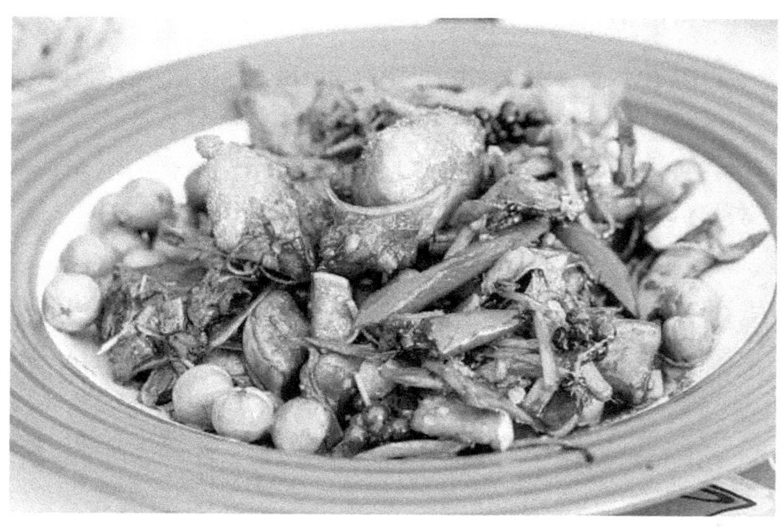

Quinoa and Vegetable Bowl

Ingredients:

For the Quinoa:

- 1 cup quinoa, rinsed and drained
- 2 cups water or vegetable broth
- Salt to taste

For the Vegetable Bowl:

- 2 cups mixed vegetables (e.g., broccoli, bell peppers, carrots, zucchini)
- 2 tablespoons olive oil
- 2 cloves garlic, minced
- 1 teaspoon dried herbs (e.g., thyme, rosemary, or oregano)
- Salt and pepper to taste

For the Dressing:

- 3 tablespoons extra-virgin olive oil
- 2 tablespoons balsamic vinegar
- 1 teaspoon Dijon mustard
- Salt and pepper to taste

Optional Toppings:

- Crumbled feta cheese

- Chopped fresh herbs (e.g., parsley, basil, or cilantro)
- Toasted nuts or seeds (e.g., almonds, sunflower seeds)

Instructions:

Quinoa:

1. In a medium saucepan, bring 2 cups of water or vegetable broth to a boil.

2. Add the rinsed quinoa and a pinch of salt. Stir, reduce heat to low, cover, and simmer for about 15-20 minutes or until the liquid is absorbed, and the quinoa is fluffy.

3. Remove from heat and let it sit, covered, for an additional 5 minutes. Fluff with a fork and set aside.

Vegetable Bowl:

1. Preheat your oven to 425°F (220°C).

2. In a large mixing bowl, combine the mixed vegetables, olive oil, minced garlic, dried herbs, salt, and pepper. Toss to coat the vegetables evenly.

3. Spread the seasoned vegetables on a baking sheet in a single layer.

4. Roast in the preheated oven for about 20-25 minutes or until the vegetables are tender and slightly caramelized. Toss them once or twice during roasting for even cooking.

Dressing:

1. In a small bowl, whisk together the extra-virgin olive oil, balsamic vinegar, Dijon mustard, salt, and pepper.

2. Taste and adjust the seasonings to your preference.

Assembly:

1. In serving bowls, start with a base of cooked quinoa.

2. Top the quinoa with the roasted vegetables.

3. Drizzle the dressing over the vegetables and quinoa.

4. Add any optional toppings, like crumbled feta cheese, fresh herbs, or toasted nuts or seeds.

5. Serve your quinoa and vegetable bowl warm.

Benefits:

- High in protein: Quinoa is a complete protein source.

- Rich in fiber: Quinoa and mixed vegetables provide dietary fiber for digestion.

- Nutrient-packed: A variety of vegetables offer a range of vitamins and minerals.

- Healthy fats: Olive oil and nuts or seeds contribute heart-healthy fats.

- Customizable: You can adapt the vegetables and toppings to your preferences.

Applications:

- A nutritious and versatile main course for lunch or dinner.

- Perfect for meal prep and can be enjoyed as a cold salad.

- Customize the vegetables based on seasonal availability.

- Suitable for vegetarians and vegans.

- This recipe can be adapted to fit various dietary preferences and restrictions.

- Use the dressing as a marinade for grilled protein like chicken or tofu.

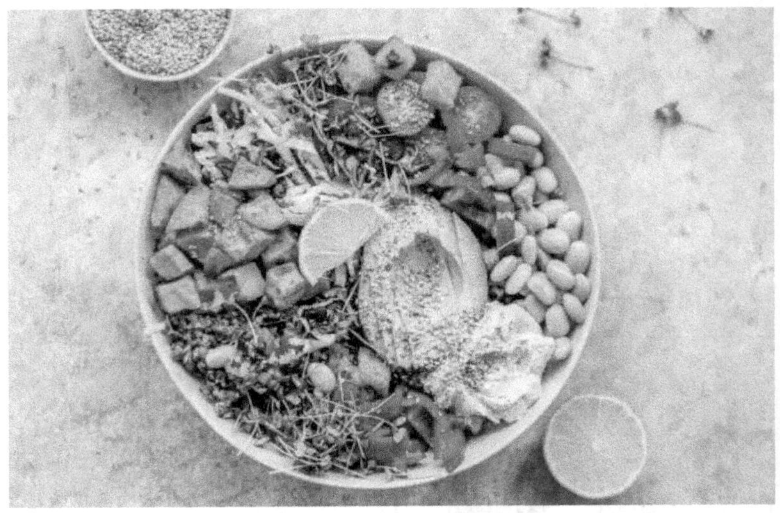

Grilled Shrimp Skewers

Ingredients:

- 1 pound large shrimp, peeled and deveined
- 2 tablespoons olive oil
- 2 cloves garlic, minced
- 1 teaspoon paprika
- 1/2 teaspoon dried oregano
- Salt and pepper to taste
- Wooden skewers, soaked in water for 30 minutes (or use metal skewers)
- Lemon wedges and fresh parsley for garnish (optional)

Instructions:

1. In a mixing bowl, combine the olive oil, minced garlic, paprika, dried oregano, salt, and pepper. Mix well to create a marinade.

2. Add the peeled and deveined shrimp to the marinade. Toss to coat the shrimp evenly. Let them marinate for about 15-20 minutes in the refrigerator.

3. Preheat your grill to medium-high heat.

4. Thread the marinated shrimp onto the soaked wooden skewers (or metal skewers if you prefer).

5. Grill the shrimp skewers for approximately 2-3 minutes per side, or until they turn pink and slightly charred.

6. Remove the shrimp from the grill.

7. Garnish with lemon wedges and fresh parsley, if desired.

Benefits:

- High-quality protein: Shrimp is a low-fat source of protein.

- Low in saturated fat: Grilled shrimp is relatively low in unhealthy saturated fats.

- Quick cooking: Shrimp cook very quickly, making this a fast and convenient meal option.

- Versatile: You can customize the marinade with your favorite seasonings and spices.

- Provides essential nutrients: Shrimp is a good source of vitamins and minerals, including selenium and vitamin B12.

Applications:

- Serve as a delicious and protein-rich main dish for a light dinner.

- Ideal for grilling at barbecues, picnics, or outdoor gatherings.

- You can use different marinades and seasonings to create various flavor profiles.

- Great as an appetizer for parties or as part of a surf and turf meal.

- Pair with a fresh salad, rice, or quinoa for a complete meal.

- Leftover grilled shrimp can be used in salads, tacos, or wraps.

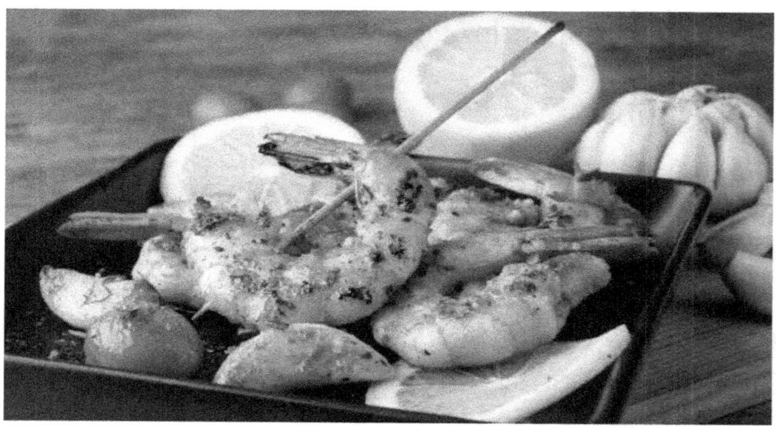

Zucchini Noodles with Pesto

Ingredients:

For the Zucchini Noodles:

- 4 medium zucchinis
- 1 tablespoon olive oil
- Salt and pepper to taste

For the Pesto Sauce:

- 2 cups fresh basil leaves, packed
- 1/2 cup grated Parmesan cheese
- 1/2 cup pine nuts or walnuts, toasted
- 2 cloves garlic, minced
- 1/2 cup extra-virgin olive oil
- Salt and pepper to taste
- Juice of 1/2 lemon (optional)

Instructions:

Pesto Sauce:

1. In a food processor, combine the basil, grated Parmesan cheese, toasted pine nuts or walnuts, and minced garlic. Pulse until the ingredients are well combined and finely chopped.

2. With the food processor running, gradually add the extra-virgin olive oil in a steady stream until the pesto becomes a smooth sauce. You may need to scrape down the sides of the bowl.

3. Add salt and pepper to taste. You can also add a squeeze of lemon juice for a bit of zing, if desired.

4. Taste the pesto and adjust the seasoning according to your preference.

Zucchini Noodles:

1. Using a spiralizer or a julienne peeler, turn the zucchinis into noodles.

2. Heat the olive oil in a large skillet over medium heat. Add the zucchini noodles and sauté for 2-3 minutes, or until they are just tender but still crisp.

3. Season the zucchini noodles with salt and pepper.

4. Remove the skillet from heat.

Assembly:

1. Toss the sautéed zucchini noodles with the prepared pesto sauce. You can use as much or as little pesto as you prefer.

2. Serve the Zucchini Noodles with Pesto immediately, garnished with extra grated Parmesan cheese and fresh basil leaves if desired.

Benefits:

- Low in carbohydrates: Zucchini noodles are a low-carb alternative to traditional pasta.

- Nutrient-dense: Zucchini is a good source of vitamins and fiber.

- Healthy fats: Nuts and olive oil in the pesto provide heart-healthy fats.

- Fresh and flavorful: The basil-based pesto is bursting with fresh herbs and garlic.

Applications:

- Ideal for a quick and healthy lunch or dinner option.

- Perfect for those following a low-carb or gluten-free diet.

- Customize the pesto with additional ingredients like sun-dried tomatoes, spinach, or arugula.

- Add grilled chicken, shrimp, or tofu for extra protein.

- Serve as a side dish or as a cold salad for picnics and potlucks.

- Make a larger batch of pesto and store it for use as a sauce on pasta, sandwiches, or as a dip.

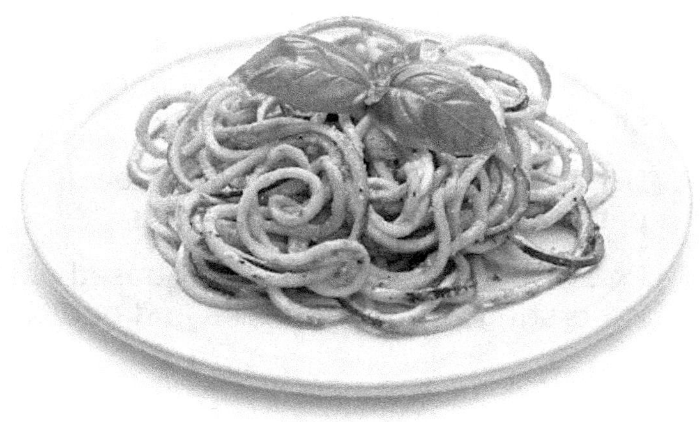

Tofu and Vegetable Curry

Ingredients:

For the Curry:

- 1 block (14 oz) extra-firm tofu, cubed

- 2 tablespoons vegetable oil

- 1 onion, finely chopped

- 2 cloves garlic, minced

- 1-inch piece of fresh ginger, minced

- 2 tablespoons curry paste (red, green, or yellow, based on your preference)

- 1 can (14 oz) coconut milk

- 1 cup vegetable broth

- 2 cups mixed vegetables (e.g., bell peppers, carrots, broccoli, and peas)

- Salt and pepper to taste

- Fresh cilantro leaves for garnish (optional)

For the Spice Blend (adjust to your heat preference):

- 1 teaspoon ground turmeric

- 1 teaspoon ground cumin

- 1 teaspoon ground coriander

- 1/2 teaspoon cayenne pepper (optional, for spiciness)

Instructions:

Tofu Preparation:

1. Press the tofu to remove excess water. You can do this by wrapping the tofu block in a clean kitchen towel and placing something heavy (like a cast-iron skillet) on top. Leave it for about 15-20 minutes, then cube the tofu.

2. In a large skillet or wok, heat 1 tablespoon of vegetable oil over medium-high heat.

3. Add the tofu cubes and cook until they are lightly browned on all sides, about 5-7 minutes. Remove the tofu from the skillet and set it aside.

Curry:

1. In the same skillet or wok, heat the remaining 1 tablespoon of vegetable oil over medium heat.

2. Add the chopped onion and cook until it becomes translucent, about 2-3 minutes.

3. Stir in the minced garlic and ginger, and cook for an additional minute until fragrant.

4. Add the curry paste and spice blend. Cook, stirring, for about 1-2 minutes to release the flavors.

5. Pour in the coconut milk and vegetable broth, stirring to combine. Bring the mixture to a simmer.

6. Add the mixed vegetables and let them cook in the curry sauce for about 10 minutes, or until they are tender.

7. Return the cooked tofu to the skillet and gently stir to combine. Allow it to heat through for another 2-3 minutes.

8. Season with salt and pepper to taste.

Assembly:

1. Serve the Tofu and Vegetable Curry hot, garnished with fresh cilantro leaves if desired.

Benefits:

- Plant-based protein: Tofu is a great source of vegetarian protein.

- Nutrient-rich: Mixed vegetables offer vitamins and fiber.

- Flavorful and aromatic: The curry paste and spices add depth to the dish.

- Vegan-friendly: This recipe is suitable for vegans and vegetarians.

- Customizable: You can adjust the spice level by modifying the curry paste and spice blend.

Applications:

- Serve the Tofu and Vegetable Curry with rice, quinoa, or naan bread for a complete meal.

- Great for a satisfying and aromatic dinner option.

- Suitable for batch cooking and meal prep.

- Customize the vegetable selection based on your preferences and what's in season.

- Leftovers can be enjoyed for lunch or dinner the next day.

- Ideal for those looking to explore and enjoy the flavors of Asian cuisine.

Turkey and Avocado Lettuce Wraps

Ingredients:

- 1 pound ground turkey
- 2 tablespoons olive oil
- 1 small onion, finely chopped
- 2 cloves garlic, minced
- 1 teaspoon ground cumin
- 1/2 teaspoon chili powder
- 1/2 teaspoon paprika
- Salt and pepper to taste
- 1 large head of iceberg or butter lettuce, leaves separated and washed
- 1 ripe avocado, sliced
- 1 tomato, diced
- 1/2 cup shredded cheese (e.g., cheddar, Monterey Jack, or a dairy-free alternative)
- Fresh cilantro leaves for garnish (optional)
- Salsa or hot sauce for serving (optional)

Instructions:

1. In a large skillet, heat the olive oil over medium-high heat.

2. Add the chopped onion and cook until it becomes translucent, about 2-3 minutes.

3. Stir in the minced garlic and cook for another minute until fragrant.

4. Add the ground turkey to the skillet and cook, breaking it apart as it browns. Cook until the turkey is no longer pink, about 5-7 minutes.

5. Season the turkey with ground cumin, chili powder, paprika, salt, and pepper. Mix well to evenly coat the meat and spices.

6. Reduce the heat to low and let the turkey simmer for an additional 2-3 minutes.

7. Remove the skillet from heat.

Assembly:

1. Spoon the seasoned ground turkey mixture into the individual lettuce leaves.

2. Top each lettuce leaf with avocado slices, diced tomato, and shredded cheese.

3. Garnish with fresh cilantro leaves if desired.

4. Serve the Turkey and Avocado Lettuce Wraps with salsa or hot sauce for added flavor, if desired.

Benefits:

- Lean protein: Ground turkey is a good source of protein with less saturated fat.

- Low in carbohydrates: Lettuce serves as a low-carb alternative to tortillas or bread.

- Healthy fats: Avocado provides monounsaturated fats and essential nutrients.

- Nutrient-rich: Tomatoes and herbs add vitamins and minerals.

- Gluten-free: Suitable for those with gluten sensitivities.

Applications:

- Ideal for a low-carb, gluten-free, or keto-friendly meal.

- Great for a quick and light lunch or dinner option.

- Customize the toppings with your favorite vegetables and condiments.

- Suitable for a family-friendly meal that's easy to prepare.

- Serve at picnics, parties, or as an appetizer at gatherings.

- These lettuce wraps can be made with different proteins such as chicken or tofu.

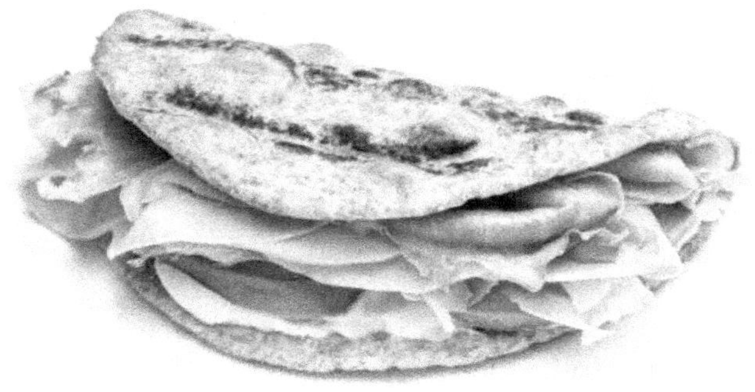

Cauliflower Rice Stir-Fry

Ingredients:

For the Cauliflower Rice:

- 1 head of cauliflower, washed and cut into florets
- 1 tablespoon vegetable oil
- Salt and pepper to taste

For the Stir-Fry:

- 2 tablespoons vegetable oil
- 2 cloves garlic, minced
- 1-inch piece of fresh ginger, minced
- 1 cup mixed vegetables (e.g., bell peppers, carrots, broccoli, and snap peas)
- 1 cup protein of your choice (e.g., tofu, chicken, shrimp, or beef)
- 3 tablespoons low-sodium soy sauce (or tamari for a gluten-free option)
- 1 tablespoon oyster sauce (optional)
- 1/2 teaspoon sesame oil
- Optional garnishes: chopped green onions, sesame seeds, chopped cilantro

Instructions:

Cauliflower Rice:

1. Place the cauliflower florets in a food processor.

2. Pulse the cauliflower until it reaches a rice-like consistency. Be careful not to overprocess, as you don't want it to become mushy.

3. Heat 1 tablespoon of vegetable oil in a large skillet or wok over medium heat.

4. Add the cauliflower rice and cook for 5-7 minutes, stirring frequently, until it becomes tender and slightly browned.

5. Season with salt and pepper to taste. Remove from the skillet and set aside.

Stir-Fry:

1. In the same skillet or wok, heat 2 tablespoons of vegetable oil over medium-high heat.

2. Add the minced garlic and ginger, and stir-fry for about 1-2 minutes until fragrant.

3. Add the protein of your choice and cook until it's no longer pink and cooked through.

4. Add the mixed vegetables and continue to stir-fry for 3-4 minutes until they are tender-crisp.

5. In a small bowl, combine the low-sodium soy sauce, oyster sauce (if using), and sesame oil.

6. Pour the sauce mixture over the stir-fry and toss to coat the ingredients evenly.

Assembly:

1. Divide the cauliflower rice into serving plates.

2. Top the cauliflower rice with the stir-fry mixture.

3. Garnish with chopped green onions, sesame seeds, and chopped cilantro if desired.

Benefits:

- Low in carbohydrates: Cauliflower rice is a low-carb substitute for traditional rice.

- Packed with vegetables: The stir-fry includes a variety of colorful and nutrient-rich veggies.

- Customizable: You can choose your preferred protein and vegetables.

- A healthy alternative: Lower in calories and carbohydrates compared to traditional stir-fry dishes.

- Suitable for gluten-free and keto diets.

Applications:

- Ideal for a low-carb and healthier version of a classic stir-fry.

- Great for those looking to incorporate more vegetables into their meals.

- Perfect for a quick weeknight dinner option.

- Customizable to your taste with different proteins and sauces.

- Make a large batch for meal prep and enjoy it as leftovers.

- Suitable for those following gluten-free or keto diets.

Greek Salad with Grilled Chicken

Ingredients:

For the Grilled Chicken:

- 2 boneless, skinless chicken breasts
- 2 tablespoons olive oil
- 2 cloves garlic, minced
- 1 teaspoon dried oregano
- Salt and pepper to taste
- Juice of 1 lemon

For the Greek Salad:

- 2 cups diced cucumbers
- 2 cups diced tomatoes
- 1 cup diced red onion
- 1 cup diced bell peppers (green, red, or yellow)
- 1 cup Kalamata olives, pitted
- 1 cup feta cheese, crumbled
- 1/4 cup fresh parsley, chopped
- 1/4 cup fresh mint leaves, chopped (optional)

For the Dressing:

- 1/4 cup extra-virgin olive oil
- 2 tablespoons red wine vinegar
- 1 teaspoon dried oregano
- Salt and pepper to taste
- Juice of 1 lemon

Instructions:

Grilled Chicken:

1. In a bowl, combine olive oil, minced garlic, dried oregano, salt, pepper, and lemon juice to make a marinade.

2. Place the chicken breasts in a resealable plastic bag or a shallow dish, and pour the marinade over them. Seal the bag or cover the dish and refrigerate for at least 30 minutes or up to 4 hours.

3. Preheat your grill to medium-high heat.

4. Remove the chicken from the marinade and grill for about 6-8 minutes per side, or until the chicken is cooked through and has nice grill marks. The internal temperature should reach 165°F (74°C).

5. Remove the chicken from the grill and let it rest for a few minutes before slicing it.

Greek Salad:

1. In a large bowl, combine the diced cucumbers, tomatoes, red onion, bell peppers, Kalamata olives, crumbled feta cheese, parsley, and optional mint leaves.

2. Toss the salad ingredients together to combine.

Dressing:

1. In a small bowl, whisk together the extra-virgin olive oil, red wine vinegar, dried oregano, salt, pepper, and lemon juice.

2. Pour the dressing over the Greek salad and toss to coat the vegetables and cheese evenly.

Assembly:

1. Divide the Greek salad among serving plates.

2. Top each salad with slices of grilled chicken.

3. Serve the Greek Salad with Grilled Chicken immediately.

Benefits:

- High-quality protein: Grilled chicken is a lean source of protein.

- Nutrient-packed: The Greek salad offers a variety of vitamins and minerals from fresh vegetables.

- Healthy fats: Olive oil provides heart-healthy monounsaturated fats.

- Fresh and flavorful: The combination of herbs, olives, and feta cheese gives this salad a burst of Mediterranean flavors.

Applications:

- Ideal for a light and nutritious lunch or dinner option.

- Perfect for warm-weather meals and outdoor gatherings.

- You can customize the salad with additional ingredients like artichoke hearts or roasted red peppers.

- Serve with pita bread or as a side dish to grilled meats.

- Suitable for those following a Mediterranean or low-carb diet.

- Make a larger batch for meal prep and enjoy it throughout the week.

Quinoa Stuffed Bell Peppers

Ingredients:

- 4 large bell peppers (any color)
- 1 cup quinoa, rinsed and drained
- 2 cups vegetable broth (or water)
- 1 tablespoon olive oil
- 1 small onion, finely chopped
- 2 cloves garlic, minced
- 1 cup mixed vegetables (e.g., carrots, corn, peas)
- 1 can (14 oz) diced tomatoes, drained
- 1 cup black beans, cooked and drained
- 1 teaspoon ground cumin
- 1/2 teaspoon chili powder
- Salt and pepper to taste
- 1 cup shredded cheese (optional, for topping)
- Fresh parsley or cilantro leaves for garnish (optional)

Instructions:

1. Preheat your oven to 375°F (190°C).

2. Cut the tops off the bell peppers, remove the seeds and membranes, and set them aside. If the bell peppers don't stand upright, you can trim the bottoms slightly to create a stable base.

3. In a medium saucepan, combine the rinsed quinoa and vegetable broth (or water). Bring to a boil, then reduce the heat, cover, and simmer for about 15-20 minutes, or until the quinoa is cooked and the liquid is absorbed. Remove from heat and fluff with a fork.

4. In a large skillet, heat the olive oil over medium heat.

5. Add the chopped onion and cook until it becomes translucent, about 2-3 minutes.

6. Stir in the minced garlic and cook for another minute until fragrant.

7. Add the mixed vegetables and cook for about 5 minutes, or until they are tender.

8. Mix in the diced tomatoes, black beans, ground cumin, chili powder, salt, and pepper. Cook for a few minutes until the mixture is heated through.

9. Add the cooked quinoa to the skillet and stir to combine all the ingredients.

10. Stuff each bell pepper with the quinoa and vegetable mixture, packing it tightly.

11. If desired, top each stuffed pepper with shredded cheese.

12. Place the stuffed peppers in a baking dish.

13. Cover the baking dish with foil and bake for 30-35 minutes, or until the peppers are tender.

14. Remove the foil and bake for an additional 5-10 minutes, or until the cheese is melted and bubbly.

Benefits:

- High in protein: Quinoa and black beans provide a good source of vegetarian protein.

- Nutrient-rich: A variety of vegetables offer vitamins and minerals.

- Fiber-filled: Quinoa and black beans contribute dietary fiber for digestion.

- A balanced meal with grains, protein, and veggies.

- Suitable for vegetarians and can be customized to be vegan.

Applications:

- A satisfying and wholesome vegetarian or vegan main course.

- Great for family dinners or when entertaining guests.

- Make it ahead and reheat for a quick weekday meal.

- Serve with a side salad or as part of a larger meal.

- Leftover filling can be used for stuffed zucchinis, tomatoes, or as a burrito filling.

- Ideal for those following a plant-based or meatless diet.

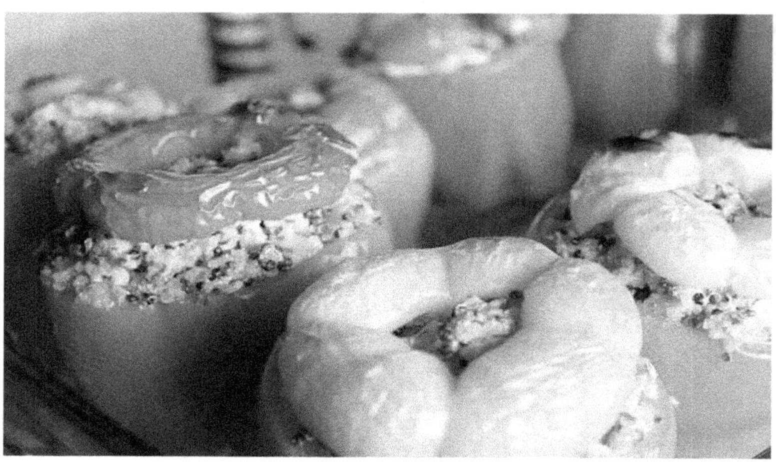

Baked Cod with Lemon and Herbs

Ingredients:

- 4 cod fillets (6-8 oz each)
- 2 tablespoons olive oil
- 2 cloves garlic, minced
- 2 tablespoons fresh lemon juice
- Zest of 1 lemon
- 1 teaspoon dried oregano
- 1 teaspoon dried thyme
- Salt and pepper to taste
- Fresh herbs for garnish (e.g., fresh parsley or dill)
- Lemon slices for garnish

Instructions:

1. Preheat your oven to 375°F (190°C).

2. In a small bowl, combine the olive oil, minced garlic, fresh lemon juice, lemon zest, dried oregano, dried thyme, salt, and pepper to create a marinade.

3. Place the cod fillets in a baking dish large enough to hold them in a single layer.

4. Pour the marinade over the cod fillets, making sure they are well-coated.

5. Cover the baking dish with foil and let the cod marinate for about 15-20 minutes at room temperature.

6. Bake the cod in the preheated oven for approximately 15-20 minutes, or until the fish flakes easily with a fork and is opaque in the center.

7. If you like, you can broil the cod for an additional 2-3 minutes at the end to brown the top slightly.

8. Garnish with fresh herbs and lemon slices.

Benefits:

- High-quality protein: Cod is a lean source of protein.

- Healthy fats: Olive oil provides heart-healthy monounsaturated fats.

- Fresh and flavorful: The combination of lemon and herbs adds brightness and depth to the dish.

- Low in carbohydrates: Suitable for low-carb and keto diets.

- Suitable for a variety of dietary preferences, including paleo and gluten-free.

Applications:

- Ideal for a quick and healthy dinner option.

- Perfect for those who enjoy the flavors of Mediterranean cuisine.

- Pair with a side of steamed vegetables or a salad for a balanced meal.

- Serve the cod over a bed of cooked quinoa or brown rice.

- Great for a weeknight meal when you need something fast and delicious.

- Can be easily adapted to suit various dietary preferences and restrictions.

Turkey and Vegetable Skillet

Ingredients:

- 1 pound ground turkey
- 2 tablespoons olive oil
- 1 small onion, chopped
- 2 cloves garlic, minced
- 1 bell pepper, diced
- 1 zucchini, diced
- 1 cup cherry tomatoes, halved
- 1 cup fresh spinach or kale
- 1 teaspoon dried oregano
- 1/2 teaspoon dried basil
- Salt and pepper to taste
- Grated Parmesan cheese for garnish (optional)

Instructions:

1. In a large skillet, heat the olive oil over medium-high heat.

2. Add the chopped onion and cook until it becomes translucent, about 2-3 minutes.

3. Stir in the minced garlic and cook for an additional minute until fragrant.

4. Add the ground turkey to the skillet and cook, breaking it apart as it browns. Cook until the turkey is no longer pink, about 5-7 minutes.

5. Season the turkey with dried oregano, dried basil, salt, and pepper. Mix well to evenly coat the meat and spices.

6. Push the cooked turkey to one side of the skillet and add the diced bell pepper and zucchini to the other side. Sauté for about 3-4 minutes, or until they begin to soften.

7. Stir in the cherry tomatoes and continue to cook for an additional 2-3 minutes, or until they are slightly softened.

8. Add the fresh spinach or kale and stir until wilted.

Benefits:

- Lean protein: Ground turkey is a lean source of protein.

- Nutrient-rich: A variety of vegetables offer vitamins, minerals, and fiber.

- Low in carbohydrates: Ideal for low-carb or keto diets.

- Quick and easy: This dish comes together in under 30 minutes.

- Versatile: You can customize the vegetables based on your preferences.

Applications:

- Ideal for a quick and healthy weeknight dinner.

- Great for a low-carb, gluten-free, or keto-friendly meal.

- Serve over cooked quinoa, rice, or pasta for a heartier meal.

- Customize with your favorite vegetables or herbs.

- Make extra for meal prep and enjoy leftovers for lunch.

- Suitable for those following various dietary preferences and restrictions.

Spaghetti Squash with Turkey Bolognese

Ingredients:

For the Spaghetti Squash:

- 1 medium spaghetti squash
- 1 tablespoon olive oil
- Salt and pepper to taste

For the Turkey Bolognese Sauce:

- 1 pound ground turkey
- 1 tablespoon olive oil
- 1 small onion, chopped
- 2 cloves garlic, minced
- 1 carrot, finely diced
- 1 celery stalk, finely diced
- 1 can (14 oz) crushed tomatoes
- 1/2 cup tomato sauce
- 1 teaspoon dried basil
- 1 teaspoon dried oregano
- Salt and pepper to taste
- Fresh basil leaves for garnish (optional)

- Grated Parmesan cheese for garnish (optional)

Instructions:

Spaghetti Squash:

1. Preheat your oven to 375°F (190°C).

2. Cut the spaghetti squash in half lengthwise and scoop out the seeds and stringy flesh.

3. Brush the cut sides of the squash with olive oil and season with salt and pepper.

4. Place the squash halves, cut side down, on a baking sheet.

5. Roast in the preheated oven for 35-45 minutes, or until the squash is tender and easily pierced with a fork.

6. Remove the squash from the oven and let it cool slightly.

7. Use a fork to scrape the flesh of the spaghetti squash into "noodles."

Turkey Bolognese Sauce:

1. In a large skillet, heat the olive oil over medium-high heat.

2. Add the chopped onion and cook until it becomes translucent, about 2-3 minutes.

3. Stir in the minced garlic, diced carrot, and diced celery. Cook for an additional 2-3 minutes, until the vegetables soften.

4. Add the ground turkey to the skillet and cook, breaking it apart as it browns. Cook until the turkey is no longer pink, about 5-7 minutes.

5. Season the turkey and vegetables with dried basil, dried oregano, salt, and pepper. Mix well to evenly coat the ingredients.

6. Stir in the crushed tomatoes and tomato sauce. Bring the mixture to a simmer, then reduce the heat and let it simmer for about 15-20 minutes, allowing the flavors to meld and the sauce to thicken.

Assembly:

1. Serve the spaghetti squash "noodles" on plates or in bowls.

2. Top with the turkey Bolognese sauce.

3. Garnish with fresh basil leaves and grated Parmesan cheese if desired.

Benefits:

- Low-carb alternative: Spaghetti squash replaces traditional pasta, making this dish lower in carbohydrates.

- Lean protein: Ground turkey is a lean source of protein.

- Nutrient-rich: Carrots and celery offer vitamins, minerals, and fiber.

- Customizable: You can adjust the seasonings and vegetables to suit your taste.

Applications:

- Ideal for a healthier version of classic spaghetti and meat sauce.

- Perfect for those following a low-carb or gluten-free diet.

- Serve as a complete meal or with a side salad.

- Make a double batch and freeze the extra Bolognese sauce for later use.

- Suitable for a family-friendly dinner or for meal prep.

Mediterranean Chickpea Salad

Ingredients:

For the Salad:

- 2 cans (15 oz each) chickpeas, drained and rinsed
- 1 cup cherry tomatoes, halved
- 1 cucumber, diced
- 1/2 red onion, finely chopped
- 1/2 cup Kalamata olives, pitted and sliced
- 1/2 cup feta cheese, crumbled (optional)
- 1/4 cup fresh parsley, chopped
- 1/4 cup fresh mint leaves, chopped (optional)

For the Dressing:

- 1/4 cup extra-virgin olive oil
- 2 tablespoons red wine vinegar
- 1 clove garlic, minced
- 1 teaspoon dried oregano
- Salt and pepper to taste
- Juice of 1 lemon (optional)

Instructions:

1. In a large mixing bowl, combine the chickpeas, halved cherry tomatoes, diced cucumber, finely chopped red onion, Kalamata olives, and crumbled feta cheese (if using).

2. In a small bowl, whisk together the extra-virgin olive oil, red wine vinegar, minced garlic, dried oregano, salt, and pepper to create the dressing.

3. Pour the dressing over the salad and toss to coat the ingredients evenly. If desired, squeeze the juice of one lemon over the salad for added flavor.

4. Add the chopped fresh parsley and mint leaves (if using) to the salad and gently toss again.

5. Let the salad sit for about 10-15 minutes to allow the flavors to meld.

Benefits:

- High in protein and fiber: Chickpeas provide a good source of plant-based protein and fiber.

- Rich in vitamins and minerals: Tomatoes, cucumbers, and fresh herbs offer a variety of nutrients.

- Healthy fats: Extra-virgin olive oil provides heart-healthy monounsaturated fats.

- Versatile and customizable: You can adjust the salad ingredients and dressing to suit your taste.

- Suitable for vegetarians and can be customized to be vegan.

Applications:

- Ideal for a light and refreshing lunch or dinner option.

- Perfect for picnics, potlucks, and as a side dish for barbecues.

- Serve as part of a Mediterranean-inspired meal with grilled meats or fish.

- Make a larger batch for meal prep and enjoy it throughout the week.

- Great for those following a vegetarian, vegan, or Mediterranean diet.

- Customize with additional ingredients like roasted red peppers or artichoke hearts.

Chicken and Broccoli Stir-Fry

Ingredients:

For the Stir-Fry:

- 2 boneless, skinless chicken breasts, thinly sliced
- 2 tablespoons vegetable oil
- 1 small onion, finely chopped
- 2 cloves garlic, minced
- 1 bunch broccoli, cut into florets
- 1 red bell pepper, thinly sliced
- 1 cup snap peas or snow peas
- 1 carrot, thinly sliced
- 1/2 cup chicken broth
- Salt and pepper to taste
- Sesame seeds for garnish (optional)

For the Stir-Fry Sauce:

- 1/4 cup low-sodium soy sauce
- 2 tablespoons oyster sauce
- 1 tablespoon honey or brown sugar
- 1 teaspoon cornstarch

Instructions:

Stir-Fry Sauce:

1. In a small bowl, whisk together the low-sodium soy sauce, oyster sauce, honey (or brown sugar), and cornstarch until well combined. Set the sauce aside.

Stir-Fry:

1. In a large skillet or wok, heat 1 tablespoon of vegetable oil over high heat.

2. Add the thinly sliced chicken and stir-fry for 3-4 minutes, or until it's cooked through and no longer pink. Remove the chicken from the skillet and set it aside.

3. In the same skillet, add the remaining 1 tablespoon of vegetable oil.

4. Add the finely chopped onion and minced garlic, and stir-fry for about 1-2 minutes until fragrant.

5. Add the broccoli florets, red bell pepper, snap peas, and carrot to the skillet. Stir-fry for 4-5 minutes, or until the vegetables are tender-crisp.

6. Return the cooked chicken to the skillet and pour the stir-fry sauce over the ingredients.

7. Add the chicken broth and continue to cook, stirring, for an additional 2-3 minutes, or until the sauce thickens and coats the chicken and vegetables.

8. Season with salt and pepper to taste.

Assembly:

1. Serve the Chicken and Broccoli Stir-Fry hot, garnished with sesame seeds if desired.

Benefits:

- High-quality protein: Chicken provides a lean source of protein.

- Nutrient-packed: Broccoli, red bell pepper, and other vegetables offer vitamins, minerals, and fiber.

- Quick and easy: This dish comes together in under 30 minutes.

- Customizable: You can adjust the vegetables and sauce to suit your taste.

- Suitable for a variety of dietary preferences, including gluten-free when using tamari.

Applications:

- Ideal for a quick and healthy weeknight dinner.

- Perfect for those looking to incorporate more vegetables into their meals.

- Serve with rice, noodles, or quinoa for a complete meal.

- Great for meal prep, as leftovers can be enjoyed for lunch.

- Customize the spice level with red pepper flakes or hot sauce.

- Suitable for those following a gluten-free or low-carb diet when served with cauliflower rice or by omitting the rice or noodles.

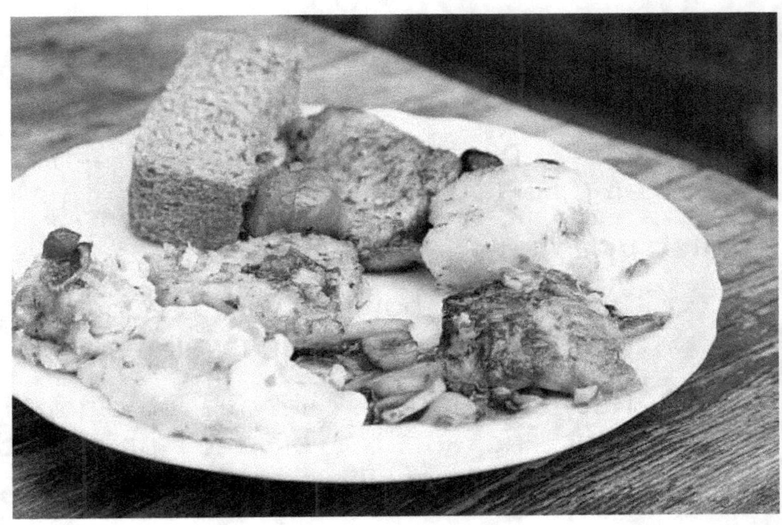

Egg White Omelette

Ingredients:

- 4 large egg whites
- 1/4 cup diced bell peppers
- 1/4 cup diced onions
- 1/4 cup diced tomatoes
- 1/4 cup diced mushrooms
- 1/4 cup diced spinach (optional)
- 1/4 cup diced lean protein (e.g., turkey, chicken, or tofu)
- 1/4 cup low-fat cheese (optional)
- 1 teaspoon olive oil or cooking spray
- Salt and pepper to taste
- Fresh herbs (e.g., chives, parsley) for garnish (optional)

Instructions:

1. In a mixing bowl, whisk the egg whites until they are frothy and well mixed.

2. Heat a non-stick skillet over medium-high heat and add the olive oil or coat the skillet with cooking spray.

3. Add the diced vegetables and lean protein to the skillet and sauté for a few minutes until they begin to soften. If you're using spinach, add it at the end, as it cooks quickly.

4. Season the vegetable mixture with salt and pepper to taste.

5. Pour the whisked egg whites over the vegetables and allow them to cook without stirring.

6. Once the edges of the omelette start to set, use a spatula to lift the edges and tilt the skillet to let the uncooked egg whites flow underneath.

7. When the omelette is mostly set but still slightly runny on top, you can optionally add low-fat cheese.

8. Carefully fold one half of the omelette over the other to create a semi-circle shape.

9. Continue to cook for a minute or two until the cheese is melted and the omelette is fully set.

10. Slide the omelette onto a plate and garnish with fresh herbs if desired.

Benefits:

- Low in calories: Egg white omelettes are lower in calories and fat compared to whole egg omelettes.

- High in protein: Egg whites are an excellent source of lean protein.

- Packed with vegetables: The omelette can include a variety of vegetables, adding vitamins and minerals.

- Customizable: You can adjust the ingredients to suit your taste and dietary preferences.

- Suitable for those looking to reduce their fat intake.

Applications:

- Ideal for a healthy and low-calorie breakfast option.

- Great for individuals focusing on weight management and protein intake.

- Serve with whole-grain toast, fruit, or a side salad for a complete meal.

- Customize with your favorite vegetables and lean protein sources.

- Suitable for those following a low-fat or low-cholesterol diet.

- Make a large batch and slice it into smaller portions for meal prep.

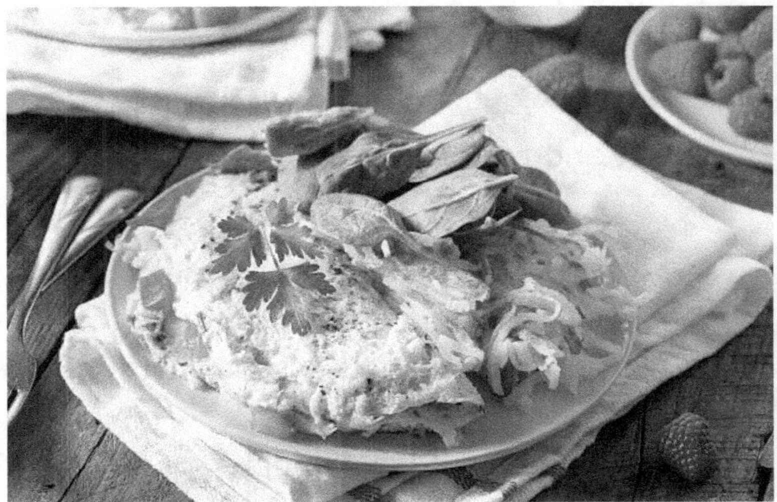

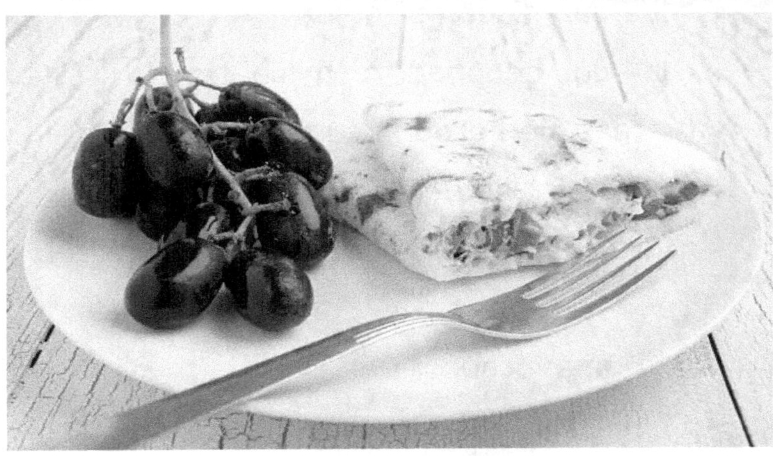

Quinoa and Black Bean Bowl

Ingredients:

For the Quinoa:

- 1 cup quinoa, rinsed and drained
- 2 cups vegetable broth (or water)
- Salt and pepper to taste

For the Black Bean Mixture:

- 1 can (15 oz) black beans, drained and rinsed
- 1 cup corn kernels (fresh, frozen, or canned)
- 1 cup diced red bell pepper
- 1/2 cup diced red onion
- 1/4 cup chopped fresh cilantro
- 1 teaspoon ground cumin
- Juice of 1 lime
- Salt and pepper to taste

For the Avocado Dressing:

- 2 ripe avocados
- 1/4 cup plain Greek yogurt (or a dairy-free alternative)

- 1 clove garlic, minced
- Juice of 1 lime
- Salt and pepper to taste
- Water (as needed to thin the dressing)

Instructions:

Quinoa:

1. In a medium saucepan, combine the quinoa and vegetable broth (or water).

2. Bring to a boil, then reduce the heat, cover, and simmer for about 15-20 minutes, or until the quinoa is cooked and the liquid is absorbed.

3. Season with salt and pepper to taste.

Black Bean Mixture:

1. In a large bowl, combine the black beans, corn kernels, diced red bell pepper, diced red onion, chopped cilantro, ground cumin, and lime juice.

2. Season with salt and pepper to taste.

3. Toss the ingredients together to create the black bean mixture.

Avocado Dressing:

1. In a food processor or blender, combine the ripe avocados, plain Greek yogurt, minced garlic, lime juice, salt, and pepper.

2. Blend until smooth. If the dressing is too thick, add a little water to achieve your desired consistency.

Assembly:

1. Divide the cooked quinoa among serving bowls.

2. Top the quinoa with the black bean mixture.

3. Drizzle the avocado dressing over the bowl.

4. Garnish with additional cilantro and lime wedges if desired.

Benefits:

- Protein-rich: Quinoa and black beans provide plant-based protein.

- High in fiber: Both quinoa and black beans are rich in dietary fiber.

- Nutrient-packed: The bowl includes a variety of vegetables and healthy fats from avocado.

- Customizable: You can adjust the ingredients and dressing to suit your taste.

- Suitable for vegetarians and can be customized to be vegan.

Applications:

- Ideal for a nutritious and satisfying lunch or dinner.

- Great for individuals looking to incorporate more plant-based protein into their diet.

- Serve as a vegetarian or vegan main course.

- Perfect for meal prep and can be enjoyed as leftovers.

- Customize with your favorite toppings like diced tomatoes, jalapeños, or grated cheese.

- Suitable for those following a vegetarian, vegan, or gluten-free diet.

CONCLUSION

As we conclude "The Endomorph Diet Cookbook," we hope you have found this culinary adventure to be both instructive and rewarding.

Our goal was to give you a cookbook that celebrates the special characteristics of the endomorph body type while simultaneously demystifying the frequently complicated realm of dieting. We hope that this journey has been fulfilling for you.

You've discovered the power of simple, quick, and individualized nutrition as you've perused these pages and recipes. You've found a long-term solution for reaching your wellness and health objectives.

Your body has experienced a steady supply of energy, your overall health has improved, and your palate has delighted in the delicious flavors that a well-planned meal can provide.

Recall that living a healthy lifestyle that allows you to be your best self is more important than simply tracking your caloric intake.

We think you can do it if you have the appropriate resources and information. The information in these pages serves as your guide, and "The Endomorph Diet Cookbook" is your tool.

We urge you to carry on with this journey as a lifetime commitment to your wellbeing rather than as a band-aid solution. Give your loved ones a taste of your newfound knowledge and allow them to reap the rewards of a diet customized to suit their own body type.

We are thrilled to have contributed to your journey toward wellbeing. Your journey has just begun and does not stop here. I hope you never stop enjoying the benefits of feeding your body, one tasty and healthful meal at a time.

We are honored that you have decided to travel with "The Endomorph Diet Cookbook" on this life-changing adventure. We hope your life is full with delicious food and good health.

www.ingramcontent.com/pod-product-compliance
Lightning Source LLC
Chambersburg PA
CBHW061003260726
48661CB00005B/2032